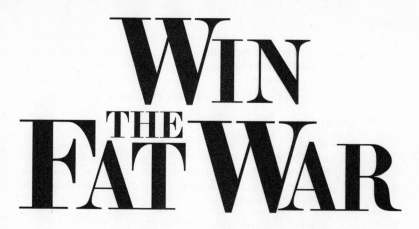

WIN THE FAT WAR

145 Real-Life Secrets to Weight-Loss Success

ANNE ALEXANDER
EDITOR-IN-CHIEF, *PREVENTION* MAGAZINE

RODALE

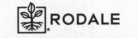

RODALE

WE INSPIRE AND ENABLE PEOPLE TO IMPROVE
THEIR LIVES AND THE WORLD AROUND THEM

*To the many friends and readers
who helped me win the fat war.*

CONTENTS

ACKNOWLEDGMENTS

This book owes a tremendous debt of gratitude—and, indeed, its origin—to the thousands of women and men who have shared their personal stories so that others can enjoy happier, healthier lives. I am grateful to all of the contributors for their honesty, authenticity, and willingness to reveal their journeys, including their dark turning points as well as the secrets that created their personal triumphs and successes. Thank you for blazing a path so that others may follow.

My sincere thanks to my editor and friend, Debora Yost, for turning this book from an idea into 256 pages of hardcover reality, with seemingly endless energy, enthusiasm, and revisions that made it better every time. Thanks also to Michele Stanten, fitness editor at *Prevention* magazine, for her time and her dedication to providing the highest quality weight-loss information and advice both in this book and in every issue of the magazine. Additional thanks to Susan Berg, who edited, shepherded, and nursed this project through its long and winding path.

Many other people had a hand in making this book a reality. For their hard work and grace under pressure, special thanks go to Susan Shelly McGovern, Doug Dollemore, Bridget Doherty, Judith Springer Riddle, Diane Gardiner Kozak, Debra L. Gordon, JoAnne Czarnecki, Margo Trott, Linda Formichelli, Therese Iknoian, and Linda Mooney.

INTRODUCTION

*I WON THE FAT WAR—
AND YOU CAN, TOO*

Congratulations! By picking up this book, you've taken the first step in a very important personal journey toward creating the life you want, free of the struggle with excess pounds, that constant battle between how you *want* to look and feel and what you see in the mirror every day.

We all come to this starting point from a different place. Maybe you're just sick and tired of feeling bad about the way you look. Maybe your doctor said that you have to get serious about your weight. Maybe you've just ridden that weight-loss roller coaster—up, up, up in pounds, down with a crash, then back up even higher next time—once too often and you want to get off for good.

Well, you can. You *can* win the fat war. Why am I so sure? Because I've been there and I won my own battle of the bulge. After nearly 10 years of being at war with my body, I finally called a ceasefire. No, I never weighed 300 pounds. Instead, like a lot of men and women, my battle was with about 20 pounds, and most of it was waged in my head.

At age 13, I discovered cellulite on my thighs and decided that I needed to lose weight *pronto*. I also made the naïve calculation that if I could change my thighs—and my body weight—I would be happy (that is, self-confident, wildly popular, all of the magic that we associate with being thin). The result was that food became the focus of my life: reward, comfort, companion, even punishment. In a way, it was simple. A "good" day was when I'd eaten only a few morsels and gallons of diet soda; a "bad" day meant that I'd slipped (how could I not?) and gorged on something from my endless list of "forbidden" foods. Instead of enjoying my life, I was focused on inane trivia like how my jeans fit at that particular nanosecond. It was a vicious cycle and a total waste of time.

Finally, after years of inner turmoil and fluctuating weight, I decided to seek the help of a supportive counselor and group of similarly obsessed women. Just meeting others who shared the same weight issues helped me see that I was far from alone.

One of the most important lessons that I learned was how to break my habit of focusing on food instead of solving the real, underlying problem. My counselor taught me how to catch myself with the simple phrase *"Stop. Slow down and think."* When I was rushing out for a box of doughnuts, this phrase would pop into my mind, and I would pause long enough to figure out what was really bothering me. Once I'd gotten to the real source of my frustration, the doughnuts became much less important. It's a simple idea, but it does the trick for me. Today, I'm pleased to report, my weight is healthy, low, and blessedly stable.

My experience with weight loss, however, was life-changing. Since then, I've been something of a crusader for healthy living. Having struggled for so long, I know what life is like on both sides—on and off the battlefield—and that it's entirely possible to win the fight once and for all.

I also know that winning isn't easy. Sometimes, it's hard work. You need to hear kind and encouraging words from people who've been in the exact same boat, to know that they've felt just as lousy as you're feeling and to know that they managed to turn things around and become who they want to be. Well, here are 145 people to tell you how they did just that.

As the editor-in-chief of the world's largest health magazine, one of my greatest pleasures is hearing success stories from readers—letters and e-mails resounding the pride and pleasure of people who finally feel really good about themselves and want to share the seemingly miraculous news that they've finally lost weight. They can run, jump, play on the floor with the kids, wear sexy clothes, feel entitled to do whatever they want.

In fact, that's the reason that I decided to create this book—to share their victories and strategies so that together we can benefit from their success. We can benefit from the inspiration and motivation that comes from knowing that, yes, when you really set your mind to it, good things *do* happen. You *can* lose weight and learn to love your body. As you'll see, their stories are filled with important life lessons for all of us.

These winners are no different from you. They're all real people, and all of them generously agreed that we could use their real names. That's a testament to their courage, because many have revealed very important personal details about their struggles and setbacks as well as their victories. But they offered to tell their full stories because they know that their honesty can truly help *you* as you make your own decisions and take the actions that are right for you.

No matter what challenges we face as individuals, I believe that all of us can use some guidance and inspiration at the beginning. To help you get started on the right foot, I've summed up these guiding principles in the "Ten Commandments of Weight Loss" in the very first chapter of this book. From the thousands of success stories that I've heard, as well as my personal experience, I am convinced that these commandments are the most important when you're trying to reach your weight-loss goals.

But I also recognize that each of us faces our individual, personal challenges. That's why I've divided the success stories into chapters that will speak most directly to you. As you'll see from their titles, the chapters focus on eating healthfully ("Feed Your Body Right"), your relationship with food ("End Emotion-Driven Eating"), exercise ("Get Your Body Moving"), self-image ("Feel Good about You"), and motivation ("Stimulate Your Determination"). If you're not sure where to begin, you might think about the issue that has been most daunting to you in the past. Maybe the stories in that chapter are the ones you want to read first!

While each story in and of itself is unique, they all share a common bond. For each person, there was a single thing—a personal experience or diet trick—that made them turn the corner to their success. These are the "Winning Actions" that you'll find featured at the end of each story. I've added my own commentary to these Winning Actions because I believe there are ways that each of us can use these actions or learn something from them as we pursue our own journeys to success.

Now—just listen to the triumphs of these winners, and let yourself be filled with possibility. All you have to do is decide that, today, you want to win the fat war.

So turn the page and embark on creating your new life.

Anne Alexander

Ten Commandments of Weight Loss

The Ten Commandments that Moses brought down from Mount Sinai can keep you on the straight and narrow in your journey through life. In much the same way, the Ten Commandments of Weight Loss can guide your weight-loss efforts and show you the way to a healthier, happier lifestyle. They'll help you get started, and they'll serve as guideposts on your personal path to success.

As you go along, some of the Ten Commandments may become more important to you than others. That's okay. Use them for inspiration and motivation.

1. Believe in Yourself

Close your eyes and take a few quiet minutes to think about what has brought you to this point in your life. Think about the reasons why *you* want to slim down, not why other people want you to. This decision is about making yourself happy, not about making others happy. Real motivation can come only from inside you.

Maybe you want to have more energy so you can go bicycling with your spouse or keep up with your kids. Maybe you want to avoid the health problems that have affected your parents or siblings. Maybe you're just tired of putting yourself down and you want to start feeling good about yourself.

Whatever reasons you come up with, write all of them down. Keep your list someplace where you'll see it often. Tape it on your medicine cabinet or attach it to the fridge. Make a copy of it for your wallet and one for your office. Read it whenever you have a few minutes. Add new reasons as you think of them.

Every time you look at your list, reaffirm your decision to lose weight. Congratulate yourself for choosing to be good to yourself. Remember that you're leaving old, unhealthy habits behind and that you're creating a new future for yourself.

Once you make the decision to feel better, to live a happier, healthier life, and to take just as good care of yourself as you do of others, you *will* succeed. Believe in yourself. Thousands of others have won the fat war. You can, too!

2. Set the Right Goals

Goals can keep you motivated and moving in the right direction—if you set the right ones. But how do you know what goals to set, and how do you make them realistic?

The first rule is to start small. Establish daily or weekly minigoals to change some aspect of your behavior that's standing between you and weight-loss success. It can be as simple as eating air-popped popcorn while you watch TV, instead of your usual potato chips. Or walking your kids to school every morning, rather than loading them into the minivan.

As you start to feel better, you'll naturally be inspired to set loftier goals. You may decide to give up potato chips completely or to increase your walking time to a half-hour or even an hour a day. It's good to keep updating your goals as you make progress, but be sure to keep them doable.

The second rule of goal setting is to write down your goals. Seeing them in front of you takes them from the abstract and makes them real. I have a friend who writes her goals on Post-It notes and sticks them on her bathroom mirror. They're the first thing that she sees every morning, and they remind her of her new priorities.

However you choose to do it, keep your goals manageable and visible. Stick with them and watch them work!

3. Eat More

Eat more to weigh less? Absolutely! You can heap your plate with juicy, sweet, wonderful-tasting fruits; colorful, crunchy vegetables; and filling, satisfying grains. Slimming down does *not* mean being hungry or skipping meals or living on iceberg lettuce and stalks of celery.

You not only can eat more, you can eat more often. Studies have shown that switching from two or three large, heavy meals to five or six healthy mini-meals keeps your metabolism revved up and burning calories. It also keeps your energy level high, so you're always ready to get up and move around.

Make your meals interesting and enticing. Try fruits and veggies that you have never had before. Many supermarkets now carry a selection of exotic produce like star fruits, Asian pears, clementines, kale, and Swiss chard. Experiment with herbs, spices, flavored vinegars, and other condiments that add tons of flavor with little fat and few calories.

Food is not the enemy when you're trying to lose weight. It's your ally. Choose wisely, and you will become slimmer, healthier, and more energized.

4. Eat Smart

Eating more can help you realize your weight-loss goals. But you have to be smart about it. If you coat your wonderful lunch salad with a high-fat dressing, it's not so wonderful anymore. If you slather your whole-grain roll with butter, it topples out of the healthy category and into the not-so-healthy one.

The easiest and fastest way to teach yourself to eat smart is to keep a food diary. In a small notebook, write down exactly when, what, and how much you eat. Was the fish broiled or fried? Did you have one serving of ice cream, or two . . . or three? Was your baked potato topped with plain low-fat yogurt and chives or with butter and sour cream?

You may be surprised at how your perception of what and how much you eat differs from what really goes into your mouth. You may never have realized how many handfuls of M&M's you grab from the office candy dish over the course of a day. Or that the bottle of cola that you drink with your lunch contains two servings rather than one. Or that your usual-size portion of fish is three times larger than it should be. All of those extra calories add up.

Learn to recognize portion sizes. Weigh and measure foods until you know what a serving looks like. And always read labels. You'll be amazed at where you'll find loads of calories lurking.

Eating smart isn't about eating boring, tasteless meals—or not eating at all. It's about eating only when you're hungry, making healthful food choices, and controlling your portions. It's about being aware of why you're eating. It's about feeding your body properly and feeling good about yourself.

5. Get Moving

An active lifestyle is extremely important for everyone, regardless of whether they want to lose weight. Time and again, studies have shown that those who exercise regularly tend to live longer and feel more satisfied with themselves than those who never get off the couch. Just think of the people that you know. Chances are that those who get out and move around regularly are more energetic and vital than those who don't.

If you're just launching an exercise program, the important thing is to start slowly. Five minutes of something as simple as walking is enough at first, especially if you've been inactive. Just increase the length of your walks by about 5 minutes a week, until you're getting 45 to 60 minutes of exercise at least 5 days a week.

This doesn't mean that you need to spend all of that time on a treadmill or stairclimber. There are dozens of activities that can provide an aerobic workout. The choice is up to you. Dust off your old 10-speed bike and go for a ride. Play a couple of sets of tennis, or sign up for an aqua-aerobics class at the local YMCA. Find an activity that you enjoy. That way, you'll be more likely to stick with it.

Also, try varying your exercise routine so that it doesn't become tedious. If you ride a stationary bike for 45 minutes on Monday, go for a walk in the woods on Tuesday. Or take your bike outside on the patio for a change of scenery. Once in a while, throw in an activity that you've never done before, like rock climbing or inline skating or tai chi.

And don't overlook the little things that you can do to enhance your health and fitness—and burn a few extra calories. Instead of driving around the supermarket parking lot three times, looking for the space closest to the door, leave your car out in the hinterlands. Clean out the garage, rake up the leaves in the yard, or hang the laundry outside rather than using the dryer.

Over time, activity and exercise will become a natural, even enjoyable part of your life. Have faith and give it a try.

6. Build Muscle

While aerobic exercise revs up your metabolism and improves your level of fitness, it's strength training that builds muscle. That's important because the more muscle you have, the higher the rate at which your body burns calories. What's more, muscle burns more calories round the clock, even when you're curled up on the couch reading a good book.

Can't imagine yourself walking into a gym and inquiring where you might find the weight room? Then do a simple but effective strength-training program in your own home, using hand weights or even soup cans. Still, you may want to consult a personal trainer, who can teach you a routine as well as proper form.

A 15- to 20-minute session, 2 or 3 days a week, is all the strength training that you need to build muscle and develop a sleeker, firmer appearance. And you'll see results in as little as 6 to 8 weeks. You'll feel stronger and more confident. Your clothes will fit better. Your belly will be flatter; your arms and legs, more toned and shapely.

So go ahead and start lifting. You'll love what you see—and how you feel.

7. Binge-Proof Your Life

If you're prone to bingeing, don't worry. You *can* stop it and take control of your eating habits. But first you must understand why it happens. What sorts of things cause you to overeat? For some people, the cause is stress, loneliness, anger, or sadness. For others, it's dining out with friends or having a good time at a party.

Reading your food diary can help you recognize and anticipate the emotions or situations that lead to your binges. As you become more aware of what's setting you off, you can avoid those situations and find other, nonfood sources of comfort.

If you feel that you are heading for a binge or if you catch yourself in the middle of one, you can still stop it. Simply walk away—leave everything where it is and get out of the house. A brisk walk around the block can give you time to think about what's making you want to eat. Once you get back home, you'll have a new perspective on the situation, and you may realize that you're not interested in eating after all.

There may be times when you're nursing a craving—say, for chocolate mocha almond ice cream—that you have no choice but to go ahead and help yourself. Not to a huge bowl, mind you. And definitely not to the whole carton. Scoop out a single serving and put the rest back in the freezer. Then really *enjoy* that ice cream. Let each spoonful melt in your mouth and wash over all of your tastebuds.

When worse comes to worst and you indulge in an all-night bingefest, don't berate yourself afterward. You have to accept what happened and move on. There's no point in kicking yourself because you messed up. Just be sure to add a half-hour to your next workout, and be extra careful about what you eat for the next few days.

8. Talk Yourself Thin

If one person on a weight-loss program is good, then one person with a partner must be better, right? In most cases, the answer is yes.

A buddy can be an encourager, a confidante, a co-conspirator, and a calming influence. She can persuade you to put on your walking shoes and go for a stroll when you'd rather be vegging out in front of the TV or pigging out at the mall. She'll listen attentively when you confess to eating a whole bag of chocolate-chip cookies, then suggest that the two of you play a couple of sets of tennis that afternoon.

So how do you go about recruiting someone for this all-important position? Use some common sense, and trust your instincts. If you run into trouble every morning at the office when the pastry cart comes around, consider asking the person in the next cubicle to be your morale booster. If you need someone to coax you out of bed for your 6:00 A.M. workout, maybe your spouse is the weight-loss partner for you.

Nobody at home with you? Look on the Internet. There are all kinds of weight-loss chat rooms, including those connected with the Web sites of organizations like Weight Watchers and Jenny Craig.

Once you think that you've found your weight-loss buddy, tell that person what you expect. Are you looking for moral support? A workout partner? Somebody to talk to when the going gets rough? Make your wants and needs clear. That's the only way that your buddy can help you.

9. Make Motivation Easy

When you first get serious about slimming down, it's easy to feel motivated. And it's a real high when you start to see results.

But after you've been plugging away at your weight-loss program for a while, it can feel a little old. Maybe you find yourself thinking, "What the heck, one doughnut won't hurt anything." Or maybe your workouts are getting on your nerves—they take up too much of your time, or they're boring. Or maybe you've reached a plateau and you haven't lost so much as an ounce in weeks.

What do you do when you hit the weight-loss skids? You jump-start your motivation, that's what.

Get out your list of reasons why you want to slim down, and remind yourself of your purpose. Remember what you weighed when you started, and note how many pounds you've lost. Count how many more minutes you can walk or run or swim. Congratulate yourself on the job that you've done so far, and adjust your goals to get you where you want to be. Be sure to write them down and put them where you'll see them.

If you haven't lost any weight for a while, try to figure out why. Maybe those doughnuts and skipped workouts have something to do with it. But if you've been faithful to your original eating-and-exercise plan, it could be that you're burning fewer calories because you weigh less. A 160-pound body burns fewer calories during a 30-minute jog than a 190-pound body. In that case, you may have to cut your calorie intake a little more or work out a little longer to make up the difference.

Keep in mind that everyone hits plateaus when they're trying to lose weight. And lapses in motivation are perfectly normal. The trick is to overcome them and move on. You've come such a long way. Don't give up now!

10. Reward Yourself

Remember when you were a kid and you brought home an excellent report card? You knew that your high grades would earn praise from your parents, and you looked forward to hearing what a good student you were. The quarters that you'd get from Grandpa weren't bad, either.

All of us like to be recognized for what we do well. This is just as true when we're trying to lose weight as when we earned an "A" in arithmetic.

Some of the most memorable rewards that you receive will come from others. But even more important are the rewards that you give yourself.

Remember the first commandment, "Believe in yourself"? When you acknowledge each weight-loss goal that you have achieved, you are honoring the commitment and hard work that you've put into creating a new, healthier life for yourself. You don't have to wait for the big, "I-lost-75-pounds!" sorts of goals, either. Something as small as adding an extra mile to your daily walk or not eating french fries for a week can be cause for celebration.

So go ahead! Take a half-day off from work. Go shopping. Get a manicure. Buy tickets to the Yankees game. Do something that you really love but don't usually make the time to do.

When you reward yourself for a job well-done, you reinforce your belief in yourself and tell yourself that you're proud of what you've accomplished. It makes you want to do more, to see how far you can go. And that's what living life to the fullest is all about.

Feed Your
Body Right

AN INSULT MADE HER FIT

A New Year's Eve party to welcome 1994 served as the wake-up call that Meredith Willson needed to get serious about slimming down.

"At the time, I weighed more than 300 pounds," recalls the 43-year-old Athens, Tennessee, resident. "Someone that I hadn't seen in years came up to me and said, 'What happened to the Meredith I used to know?' It was a shock—and shock therapy is a good way to get inspired."

The next day, Meredith set her sights on a rather lofty resolution: to lose 120 pounds in 12 months. It was ambitious, but Meredith was convinced that eliminating red meat and processed food from her diet would do the trick. "Cheese and butter were the toughest," she says. "Instead of giving them up completely, I switched to fat-free cheese and butter substitutes." She also began eating more fresh foods—fruits, vegetables, and whole grains.

Meredith read cookbooks that taught her how to make the most of fresh ingredients in her cooking. She also planted a garden chock full of organic produce, including tomatoes, squash, broccoli, asparagus, and eggplant. "The closer you get to the ground, the better off you'll be, nutrient-wise," she says. Then, using her homegrown produce plus healthful staples from the supermarket, she spent time each weekend preparing food from scratch. She even made her own pasta, tomato sauce, and baked sweet-potato chips.

Even Meredith couldn't believe how well her switch from processed foods to fresh worked. "I lost 12 pounds every month—ka-bam, ka-bam, ka-bam," she says. "I never even hit a plateau."

In just over a year, Meredith managed to take off 150 pounds. And she has maintained that weight loss ever since.

AT DINNERTIME, SHE DESERTS HER FAMILY

Make no mistake: Debbee Sereduck loves her husband and her three children. But for 3 years, she refused to eat dinner with them. Sacrificing a little family togetherness was tough, but it helped Debbee take off an astounding 234 pounds.

Debbee, a 38-year-old resident of Spokane, Washington, doesn't remember a time when she was thin. At 5 foot 11, she carried her weight well—for a while. But the scale never seemed to stop climbing upward. By age 33, she had reached 414 pounds.

Self-conscious about her appearance and concerned about the effects that her weight might have on her health, Debbee felt that she had to slim down. She just couldn't get herself motivated to do it. That changed one day in 1994, when she turned on her television and saw rescue workers extricating a large woman from her home and placing her in a special van to take her to the hospital. "The reporter mentioned that the woman weighed 560 pounds, and I was mortified," Debbee says. "That wasn't much more than I weighed."

With the image of the woman fresh in her mind, Debbee launched a self-styled weight-loss program that consisted primarily of eating low-fat foods in more sensible portions and riding a stationary bike. "I knew what I had to do," she says. "I just needed the motivation to do it."

Exercising was tough at first because Debbee was so overweight and out of shape. "I'd just tell myself, I'm going to pedal that bike for as long as I can,'" she says. "I made myself sit on it for an hour every day, whether or not I was actually riding."

Debbee had an easier time adjusting her eating habits, but dinnertime remained a struggle. How could she eat a carefully portioned meal while watching her family help themselves to seconds? How could she just throw away perfectly good food that her kids didn't finish?

Rather than wrestle with these temptations, Debbee decided to walk away from them. Every evening, she prepared dinner and served it to her family. Then she took her meal into the living room and ate by herself. She didn't return to the kitchen or dining room until everything was cleaned up and put away. "This kept me from dipping into the serving bowls for extra helpings and from finishing off the kids' uneaten food," she says. "It also gave me a few minutes of peace and quiet."

Her strategy worked like a charm. Over the next 3 years, Debbee took off 234 pounds, reaching her goal weight of 180. She has held steady ever since.

Were all of those dinners alone worth the effort? Debbee thinks so. Now that she's fit, she has even more opportunities to enjoy life with her family. "I used to be a very active person, but I hadn't been on a bicycle since I was 11 or 12. I really wanted to go riding with my kids, which we now do all the time," she says. "I'm able to do the kinds of things that I couldn't do before."

Go solo. *If being around your family at dinner tempts you to overeat, do what Debbee did and eat your meal away from temptation. You'll feel satisfied with what's on your plate and avoid the urge for seconds. As a bonus, you can even enjoy having quiet time for yourself.*

HALF HER BODY WEIGHT—GONE

At age 31, Pamela Joyce Kimrey had to face facts.

Her father had died of a massive heart attack when he was just 35 years old. Pamela Joyce wondered if the same fate awaited her. After a lifetime of overeating and almost 2 decades of yo-yo dieting, she weighed 274 pounds. And she was scared.

Pamela Joyce, of Warrenville, South Carolina, traced her seemingly endless appetite to her childhood. "When I was born, I weighed a little more than 4 pounds," she explains. "My parents left the hospital with instructions to feed me as often and as much as they could." And they did. By the time she was in fourth grade, her weight hovered around 130 pounds.

Through high school, Pamela Joyce continued to gain. She graduated weighing close to 250 pounds, far too much for her 5-foot-2 frame. "I didn't want to go through college overweight. I wanted to fit in," she recalls. "So I put myself on what I considered a diet. I ate less, but I ate poorly—mostly deep-fried, sugary, and fatty foods." Over the next year, she took off 70 pounds. "At 180 pounds, I still weighed too much for my height," she says. "But I held steady for several years, right through my wedding in March 1987."

As Pamela Joyce settled into married life, the pounds started coming back. "Twenty-five pounds stuck around after I gave birth to our only child, Houston," she says. "The rest of the weight resulted from too many meals of fried food smothered in gravy, plus thousands of calories worth of junk food and soda."

By October 1996, Pamela Joyce had reached her top weight of 274 pounds. "One night, I was lying in bed, feeling disgusted with myself. I started thinking about my dad, and I realized that I could die young if I didn't take better care of myself. It was my wake-up call."

The very next day, Pamela Joyce went to her local library and took out every nutrition, fitness, and weight-loss book that she could find. When she read them, she found three themes that came up over and over again: a low-fat diet with portion control, regular exercise, and plenty of water.

Based on the information that she had collected, Pamela Joyce put herself on a strict 1,200-calorie-a-day diet. She cut out junk food, whole milk, and butter and began grilling and baking food instead of frying it. She also invested in a kitchen scale to keep tabs on portion sizes.

Because she was accustomed to eating as much as she wanted, Pamela Joyce had to find a way to keep her stomach full throughout the day. One of her favorite tricks was to save a part of each meal for later in the day. "If my breakfast consisted of a cup of raisin bran, a half-cup of skim milk, and a banana, I'd save the banana for a mid-morning snack," she explains. "Likewise, I'd keep half of my lunch sandwich for an afternoon snack. If I ate out, I'd have half of my entrée wrapped to go before I'd even take a bite."

This strategy helped Pamela Joyce stay within her 1,200-calorie limit without feeling hungry. Between her improved eating habits, her daily workouts (alternating aerobic exercise and strength training), and her consumption of gallons of water a week, she managed to lose 137 pounds—exactly half of her body weight—in a little more than 2 years. She's been holding steady since November 1998.

"There is absolutely no way to compare the old me with the new me," Pamela Joyce says. "I could never have imagined how wonderful I feel. I can keep up with my son and not worry about embarrassing him—except maybe when we're inline skating in the park. Good health has become a way of life for me and my family."

WINNING ACTION

Eat less more often. *Three cheers for Pamela Joyce. What an incredible story! If you can't resist between-meal snacking, do what Pamela Joyce did and save part of a meal for later on. You'll never get too hungry, since you'll be feeding your body every few hours. Plus, you'll avoid taking in too many calories in one sitting.*

95 POUNDS IN 1 YEAR: WEIGHT LOSS FOR THE RECORD BOOK

For Kelly Jens, food was once an all-consuming passion.

"I was always thinking about what my next meal would be," says the 28-year-old Glenwood, Iowa, native. "When I'd go out to eat, I'd try to pick places with the biggest portions or the most courses. I especially liked Quarter Pounders with Cheese, nachos, pizza with extra cheese, and anything with Alfredo sauce."

Always on the hefty side, Kelly couldn't stop eating—or stop gaining weight. By Christmas 1997, she had reached 220 pounds. "In a picture with my husband and my two kids, my little 1-year-old looks like a doll in my huge lap," she recalls. "I thought to myself, 'I don't want my children to have a fat, unhealthy mother.'"

It was time to change her life.

Using information she gathered from *Prevention* magazine and books by weight-loss guru Richard Simmons, Kelly determined that she would need to trim her daily calorie intake to 1,400 in order to achieve and maintain a healthy weight.

Obviously, that was far fewer calories than she had been consuming. To help herself stay on course, she began keeping a food diary. Kelly would write down every morsel she ate and every drop she drank—usually before she ate or drank it. She also noted the calorie and fat content of each item.

To help herself burn calories, Kelly started using a Health Walker, a nonimpact machine that allows the legs to swing back and forth to simulate striding. At first, she worked out for 15 minutes per session, then gradually built up to an hour a day—a schedule that she still maintains. She also does strength training twice a week, exercises to a kickboxing video, and jumps rope.

In 1 year, Kelly lost 95 pounds. And the weight hasn't come back. For that, she credits her food diary. "I never really knew how much I was eating until I starting writing it down and reviewing it," she explains. "Even though I've learned what I can eat and how much, I still keep a diary. It's a good tool for helping me maintain my present weight."

WINNING ACTION

Keep a diary. *Buy a small spiral-bound notebook and carry it with you. Immediately after meals and snacks,*